LOSE 10KG IN 10 DAYS

By Nkiru Ojimadu

ISBN-10: 1548866237

Introduction

Discover the guaranteed secrets that will help you lose weight fast and keep it off (if you are determined) – without dieting or exercise – with this wonder mini book from the author of the bestseller, *Found By Mercy*

Would you like to look, feel younger and healthier than ever without long crash diets exhausting exercise?

Want to lose weight without counting calories, starving yourself, or working yourself out in the gym?

Then this book is for you! This wonder mini book will help you lose 1kd daily! Yes, you heard me right! 1 kilogram per day!

Let's dig in and find out how it works...

I was 99kg!

It Is Possible to Lose 10kg in 10 days but it won't be pure body fat.

I've tested this plan on myself and on clients who wanted to lose weight fast before an event like a book launch (in my own case) a vacation or photoshoot, and it works wonders.

I went from 99kg to 89kg here

In fact, when I or some of my

clients use this, we look like we've been on a three- or four-week diet after just one week.

Although this won't be a long-term fix, for some that can't control themselves afterwards but, this can kick-start your weight loss journey and motivate you for more sustainable long-term changes. Though it's all in your hands, you can fire yourself up to keep the weight even after the 9 - 10day course ends. by making up your mind to eat right afterwards.

However, I must repeat that it won't be easy. To come out a success from this diet, you must really, really work on your mind. If you convince your mind to be cooperative, then you will win.

It won't be easy but it is very possible. If I could, you can!

I went on this diet the 2nd time when I needed to lose weight for my first book launch.

It is a diet that anyone that wants to embark in any kind of health plan should start with. It does wonders!

The first time, I lost 10kg in 10 days! The 2nd time I lost 5kg in 9days. It is said that, the amount of kilograms you lose tend to reduce with time, when you redo the same type of diet.

 Reason being that the body gets used to it and becomes "immune" to the effects of this diet with time.

I use this diet once in a while to keep myself fit.
Later, I weighed 79kg. From 99kg to 79kg!

In the picture below, is me holding my first book "Found By Mercy". A mind blowing one!
Click on the link to get it on Okadabooks:
https://goo.gl/mlHJKe

 Or at Amazon :
https://goo.gl/Qyl26B

Do check my other books "Relationships101" and "Who's right? He said, She Said" (This last book was co-authored by my husband, Obi Ojimadu, by just typing my name - Nkiru Ojimadu on Amazon.com or at Okadabooks.com.

Many of my clients have also used this and are happy not only that they lost a great amount of weight in such a short period but they are also so happy, how cheap this diet is.

So now friends ...
Let's do this!

This 9 day Diet plan is a non-standard, modern way to effectively lose weight without compromising on health. You can lose from 8-11kg in 9days with this diet plan. The use of popular and customary products makes it possible to comfortably and painlessly lose weight without physical and psychological stress. You do not have to starve and fight the emerging desire to eat at an inopportune time.

This diet is based on the principles of healthy nutrition and knowledge of the body's needs for vitamins, minerals and beneficial microelements. It allows you not only to get rid of extra pounds but thanks to the consistent alternation of products from different groups and the consumption of large amounts of liquid, the body is thoroughly purified, immunity is strengthened and a feeling of lightness appears.

Duration of the diet is nine days, which are divided into three separate stages. I titled it, lose 10kg in 10days just to make it rhyme. However, the number of kilograms you will lose, if you are trying this for the first time varies from 8- 11 kg in 10 days and also depends on how much excess weight you have.

Each three-day stage is an independent mono-diet. Only that, three days, you will have to "enjoy" the monotonous food. The change of dishes on the fourth and seventh day brings a pleasant variety in the diet menu. For this diet plan , you will need, rice, chicken and vegetables. It's that simple.

The first stage - a three-day rice mono diet.

So, the first three days wanting to lose weight, eat **only rice,** still water and green tea. Prepared rice is simply enough. On the eve of the next day, in the evening, a glass of rice soaked in cold water, and in the morning, we pour it into boiling water and cook for no more than 15 minutes. This way of preparing the dish allows you to preserve all the most important properties of rice. For breakfast, eat a cup of cooked rice.

P.S. Wild rice is better. In fact, I used buckwheat.

The remaining amount is divided into equal parts in such a way that it will be enough for up to 7pm, when used every hour. It is not by chance that rice is the first product to lose weight in this diet.

Rice does not excite gastric secretion because it contains substances that have the properties to envelop the walls of the stomach. Having eaten an insignificant quantity of the dish prepared from rice, you will feel full. In addition, rice does not contain salt and there is no gluten in it, which can provoke allergic reactions. At the same time, dishes from rice cereals are rich in vitamins B3, PP, B1, B2, E, B6. B vitamins help to strengthen the nervous system, help to convert nutrients into energy and affect the condition of hair, skin, and nails.

Lecithin, which is found in rice, helps to improve brain activity. It is the combination of useful properties of rice that cleanses the body in the first three days of the diet.

 The second stage is a mono-diet based on chicken meat.

The main component of the next three days of the diet, the fourth, fifth and sixth, is **chicken meat**. In the ready-to-eat form, it should be cooked meat and meat, free from skins and grease. The daily portion is from 1 kg to 1.2 kg. Prepared chicken is divided into small portions and eaten throughout the day, washed down with still water or green tea ⍰.

This diet prudently applies a similar change of products in order to fill the body with missing trace elements, which are contained only in meat. It is chicken that can effectively replace pork, lamb and beef. With a low-calorie content, this is a great source of amino acids and protein. Along with vitamins C, A, E, etc., chicken meat contains iron, potassium, zinc and phosphorus. In addition, due to the large number of polyunsaturated fatty acids, chicken is considered one of the best tools for the prevention of stroke, heart attack and ischemic disease. The low content of collagen contributes to the fact that chicken meat is easily digested. This property is especially valuable for obesity, diabetes, diseases of the gastrointestinal tract. Protein, in sufficient quantity contained in chicken, is very well assimilated and has an effect on the buildup of muscle mass, cell division, the development of brain activity, the construction of bone tissues. Chicken meat in boiled form is recommended to include in almost all diets. It is especially useful for those people who carefully monitor or watch their health and weight.

P.S. - During second stage, you can also use only fish instead of chicken. When I had this diet, I used all sorts of white proteins, for example: egg white, all sorts of white fish, squid, 0% cottage cheese etc. However, you might get a better result if you stick to ONLY one product.

The Third Stage is a **vegetable mono-diet**. All that is required for the final three days of this diet are vegetables.

Daily you need 800 grams of any type of vegetables that you know and see on the shelves of the stores, fresh or boiled vegetables. Distribute portions for the whole day, up till 7pm and enjoy. A lot has been said about the benefits of vegetables. Nevertheless, in the context of this diet, it is the vegetables that will make the final touch and fill the stock of missing trace elements and nutrients.

Vegetables do not contain fats and are very rich in useful fiber. Vitamins and mineral salts provide a rush of energy and heal the entire body. This is the most accessible source of minerals and vitamins.

In dietetics, vegetables are used to speed up metabolism and quickly remove toxins from the body. Daily consumption of vegetables improve appetite and speed up metabolism by 15-20%.

Constant meals with vegetables strengthen the processes of bile formation, improves liver function and heals the intestinal microflora. A set of vitamins, essential antioxidants, minerals and trace elements found in vegetables reliably protects against diseases and strengthens immunity.

Thanks to the vegetable mono diet, strength is restored and the general condition improves. Consumption of liquid during this diet is extremely necessary. To get rid of excess weight, **drink at least 2.5 liters of water a day. If you are over 65kg of weight, drink more.** As it was repeatedly written above, for this purpose it is possible to choose mineral still water or green tea. It is permissible to mix and alternate water and tea. However, you must definitely follow certain rules when drinking. **Do not take food with water or tea.** Also, **do not drink immediately after eating**. The time between eating and drinking should be at least 45 minutes. In addition, don't drink after 5pm. **Tea should NOT be with sugar.**

In extreme cases, you can put a little honey.

P.S. - In stage three, I used only green vegetables.

Recommendations and rules

The main principle of dietetics, eat often and gradually, shows an excellent result in this diet. However, do not forget, **DO NOT ADD ANYTHING TO THE FOOD, NOTHING AT ALL. The products should be cooked and consumed without salt, sugar and spices.**

Your body will receive from the products included in the list of diets, all the necessary and useful substances. **All other add-ons that you want to include on your own in the menu, will nullify all efforts. Do not experiment.**

Yeah, do not drink alcohol during this period.
 A lot of my clients, have made use of this diet and received excellent results.

I recommend to eat the last meal not later than 7pm. Moreover, the effectiveness will greatly increase if the diet is combined with water procedures, massage and low density physical exercises.

 Issues like, weakened immunity and elementary cold can cause great and irreparable damage to the body. Do not create for yourself an artificial extreme situation. Any diet for weight loss, in this case, can become just such a "trigger" that will undermine your health.

DO NOT GO ON THIS DIET IF YOU HAVE:

1. Stomach ulcer.
2. Heart disease.
3. A cold etc.

Before you start to put your figure in order, put your health in order. Be sure to consult with your doctor about the possibility to start this procedure of losing weight.

This type of diet plan is to motivate you to start and later, continue eating healthy and be in shape even after the diet. Stir your mind up so that you do not go back to eating junk after the 9days program because if you do not hold your appetite for "sweets and their family" , "junk and his brothers" , you might end up gaining double what you lost.

To help out, make sure you read my book "Lose 10 kg in 2Months - Never Feel Hungry dieting" , it will help you maintain a good health and shape.

Can You Handle It?
Yes, you can! ♡

To maintain a great figure after this diet I would advise you to follow it up with my other book "Lose 10kg in 2 Months" on Amazon.

Nkiru Ojimadu
A Multi Award Winning Personality,
Life Transformational Coach,
Best Selling Author,
International Speaker.
Co-Founder Relationships 101.
TV Host.

Follow me on social media

Disclaimer: I am not a dietician or a medical doctor. In this writeup, I shared with you actions that I took that made me and many that I coach through the years lose tons of weight and still keep them. I went from 99kg to 74kg!

So, I suggest that before you start executing any of the plans I shared here, please consult your doctor.

www.ingramcontent.com/pod-product-compliance
Lightning Source LLC
Chambersburg PA
CBHW060343290526
45791CB00004B/1512